Personal details

Name _____ Age _____

Telephone numbers _____ / _____

Address _____

_____

Emergency contacts

Name _____

Telephone number _____

Name _____

Telephone number _____

Important information

Allergies _____

Medication _____

Antidiabetics _____

Insulin _____

Other _____

_____

_____

_____

Start of week date _____

Monday		Before	After	Dose	Notes
	Breakfast				
	Lunch				
	Dinner				
	Night				

Tuesday		Before	After	Dose	Notes
	Breakfast				
	Lunch				
	Dinner				
	Night				

Wednesday		Before	After	Dose	Notes
	Breakfast				
	Lunch				
	Dinner				
	Night				

Thursday		Before	After	Dose	Notes
	Breakfast				
	Lunch				
	Dinner				
	Night				

Notes _____
_____
_____
_____

Friday		Before	After	Dose	Notes
	Breakfast				
	Lunch				
	Dinner				
	Night				

Saturday		Before	After	Dose	Notes
	Breakfast				
	Lunch				
	Dinner				
	Night				

Sunday		Before	After	Dose	Notes
	Breakfast				
	Lunch				
	Dinner				
	Night				

Notes _____

_____

_____

_____

_____

_____

_____

_____

_____

_____

_____

_____

Start of week date _____

Monday		Before	After	Dose	Notes
	Breakfast				
	Lunch				
	Dinner				
	Night				

Tuesday		Before	After	Dose	Notes
	Breakfast				
	Lunch				
	Dinner				
	Night				

Wednesday		Before	After	Dose	Notes
	Breakfast				
	Lunch				
	Dinner				
	Night				

Thursday		Before	After	Dose	Notes
	Breakfast				
	Lunch				
	Dinner				
	Night				

Notes _____

_____

_____

_____

Friday		Before	After	Dose	Notes
	Breakfast				
	Lunch				
	Dinner				
	Night				

Saturday		Before	After	Dose	Notes
	Breakfast				
	Lunch				
	Dinner				
	Night				

Sunday		Before	After	Dose	Notes
	Breakfast				
	Lunch				
	Dinner				
	Night				

Notes _____

_____
_____
_____
_____
_____
_____
_____
_____
_____
_____

Start of week date _____

Monday		Before	After	Dose	Notes
	Breakfast				
	Lunch				
	Dinner				
	Night				

Tuesday		Before	After	Dose	Notes
	Breakfast				
	Lunch				
	Dinner				
	Night				

Wednesday		Before	After	Dose	Notes
	Breakfast				
	Lunch				
	Dinner				
	Night				

Thursday		Before	After	Dose	Notes
	Breakfast				
	Lunch				
	Dinner				
	Night				

Notes _____

_____

_____

_____

Friday		Before	After	Dose	Notes
	Breakfast				
	Lunch				
	Dinner				
	Night				

Saturday		Before	After	Dose	Notes
	Breakfast				
	Lunch				
	Dinner				
	Night				

Sunday		Before	After	Dose	Notes
	Breakfast				
	Lunch				
	Dinner				
	Night				

Notes _____
_____
_____
_____
_____
_____
_____
_____
_____
_____
_____

Start of week date _____

Monday		Before	After	Dose	Notes
	Breakfast				
	Lunch				
	Dinner				
	Night				

Tuesday		Before	After	Dose	Notes
	Breakfast				
	Lunch				
	Dinner				
	Night				

Wednesday		Before	After	Dose	Notes
	Breakfast				
	Lunch				
	Dinner				
	Night				

Thursday		Before	After	Dose	Notes
	Breakfast				
	Lunch				
	Dinner				
	Night				

Notes _____

_____

_____

_____

Friday		Before	After	Dose	Notes
	Breakfast				
	Lunch				
	Dinner				
	Night				

Saturday		Before	After	Dose	Notes
	Breakfast				
	Lunch				
	Dinner				
	Night				

Sunday		Before	After	Dose	Notes
	Breakfast				
	Lunch				
	Dinner				
	Night				

Notes _____
_____
_____
_____
_____
_____
_____
_____
_____
_____
_____

Start of week date _____

Monday		Before	After	Dose	Notes
	Breakfast				
	Lunch				
	Dinner				
	Night				

Tuesday		Before	After	Dose	Notes
	Breakfast				
	Lunch				
	Dinner				
	Night				

Wednesday		Before	After	Dose	Notes
	Breakfast				
	Lunch				
	Dinner				
	Night				

Thursday		Before	After	Dose	Notes
	Breakfast				
	Lunch				
	Dinner				
	Night				

Notes _____

_____

_____

_____

Friday		Before	After	Dose	Notes
	Breakfast				
	Lunch				
	Dinner				
	Night				

Saturday		Before	After	Dose	Notes
	Breakfast				
	Lunch				
	Dinner				
	Night				

Sunday		Before	After	Dose	Notes
	Breakfast				
	Lunch				
	Dinner				
	Night				

Notes _____
_____
_____
_____
_____
_____
_____
_____
_____
_____
_____

Start of week date _____

Monday		Before	After	Dose	Notes
	Breakfast				
	Lunch				
	Dinner				
	Night				

Tuesday		Before	After	Dose	Notes
	Breakfast				
	Lunch				
	Dinner				
	Night				

Wednesday		Before	After	Dose	Notes
	Breakfast				
	Lunch				
	Dinner				
	Night				

Thursday		Before	After	Dose	Notes
	Breakfast				
	Lunch				
	Dinner				
	Night				

Notes _____
_____
_____

Friday		Before	After	Dose	Notes
	Breakfast				
	Lunch				
	Dinner				
	Night				

Saturday		Before	After	Dose	Notes
	Breakfast				
	Lunch				
	Dinner				
	Night				

Sunday		Before	After	Dose	Notes
	Breakfast				
	Lunch				
	Dinner				
	Night				

Notes _____
_____
_____
_____
_____
_____
_____
_____
_____
_____
_____

Start of week date _____

Monday		Before	After	Dose	Notes
	Breakfast				
	Lunch				
	Dinner				
	Night				

Tuesday		Before	After	Dose	Notes
	Breakfast				
	Lunch				
	Dinner				
	Night				

Wednesday		Before	After	Dose	Notes
	Breakfast				
	Lunch				
	Dinner				
	Night				

Thursday		Before	After	Dose	Notes
	Breakfast				
	Lunch				
	Dinner				
	Night				

Notes _____

Friday		Before	After	Dose	Notes
	Breakfast				
	Lunch				
	Dinner				
	Night				

Saturday		Before	After	Dose	Notes
	Breakfast				
	Lunch				
	Dinner				
	Night				

Sunday		Before	After	Dose	Notes
	Breakfast				
	Lunch				
	Dinner				
	Night				

Notes _____

_____

_____

_____

_____

_____

_____

_____

_____

_____

_____

_____

_____

Start of week date _____

Monday		Before	After	Dose	Notes
	Breakfast				
	Lunch				
	Dinner				
	Night				

Tuesday		Before	After	Dose	Notes
	Breakfast				
	Lunch				
	Dinner				
	Night				

Wednesday		Before	After	Dose	Notes
	Breakfast				
	Lunch				
	Dinner				
	Night				

Thursday		Before	After	Dose	Notes
	Breakfast				
	Lunch				
	Dinner				
	Night				

Notes _____
_____
_____
_____

Friday		Before	After	Dose	Notes
	Breakfast				
	Lunch				
	Dinner				
	Night				

Saturday		Before	After	Dose	Notes
	Breakfast				
	Lunch				
	Dinner				
	Night				

Sunday		Before	After	Dose	Notes
	Breakfast				
	Lunch				
	Dinner				
	Night				

Notes _____
_____
_____
_____
_____
_____
_____
_____
_____
_____
_____

Start of week date _____

Monday		Before	After	Dose	Notes
	Breakfast				
	Lunch				
	Dinner				
	Night				

Tuesday		Before	After	Dose	Notes
	Breakfast				
	Lunch				
	Dinner				
	Night				

Wednesday		Before	After	Dose	Notes
	Breakfast				
	Lunch				
	Dinner				
	Night				

Thursday		Before	After	Dose	Notes
	Breakfast				
	Lunch				
	Dinner				
	Night				

Notes _____

_____

_____

_____

Friday		Before	After	Dose	Notes
	Breakfast				
	Lunch				
	Dinner				
	Night				

Saturday		Before	After	Dose	Notes
	Breakfast				
	Lunch				
	Dinner				
	Night				

Sunday		Before	After	Dose	Notes
	Breakfast				
	Lunch				
	Dinner				
	Night				

Notes _____

_____

_____

_____

_____

_____

_____

_____

_____

_____

Start of week date _____

Monday		Before	After	Dose	Notes
	Breakfast				
	Lunch				
	Dinner				
	Night				

Tuesday		Before	After	Dose	Notes
	Breakfast				
	Lunch				
	Dinner				
	Night				

Wednesday		Before	After	Dose	Notes
	Breakfast				
	Lunch				
	Dinner				
	Night				

Thursday		Before	After	Dose	Notes
	Breakfast				
	Lunch				
	Dinner				
	Night				

Notes _____

_____

_____

_____

Friday		Before	After	Dose	Notes
	Breakfast				
	Lunch				
	Dinner				
	Night				

Saturday		Before	After	Dose	Notes
	Breakfast				
	Lunch				
	Dinner				
	Night				

Sunday		Before	After	Dose	Notes
	Breakfast				
	Lunch				
	Dinner				
	Night				

Notes _____

_____
_____
_____
_____
_____
_____
_____
_____
_____
_____
_____

Start of week date _____

Monday		Before	After	Dose	Notes
	Breakfast				
	Lunch				
	Dinner				
	Night				

Tuesday		Before	After	Dose	Notes
	Breakfast				
	Lunch				
	Dinner				
	Night				

Wednesday		Before	After	Dose	Notes
	Breakfast				
	Lunch				
	Dinner				
	Night				

Thursday		Before	After	Dose	Notes
	Breakfast				
	Lunch				
	Dinner				
	Night				

Notes _____
_____
_____
_____

Friday		Before	After	Dose	Notes
	Breakfast				
	Lunch				
	Dinner				
	Night				

Saturday		Before	After	Dose	Notes
	Breakfast				
	Lunch				
	Dinner				
	Night				

Sunday		Before	After	Dose	Notes
	Breakfast				
	Lunch				
	Dinner				
	Night				

Notes _____
_____
_____
_____
_____
_____
_____
_____
_____
_____
_____
_____

Start of week date _____

Monday		Before	After	Dose	Notes
	Breakfast				
	Lunch				
	Dinner				
	Night				

Tuesday		Before	After	Dose	Notes
	Breakfast				
	Lunch				
	Dinner				
	Night				

Wednesday		Before	After	Dose	Notes
	Breakfast				
	Lunch				
	Dinner				
	Night				

Thursday		Before	After	Dose	Notes
	Breakfast				
	Lunch				
	Dinner				
	Night				

Notes _____

_____

_____

_____

Friday		Before	After	Dose	Notes
	Breakfast				
	Lunch				
	Dinner				
	Night				

Saturday		Before	After	Dose	Notes
	Breakfast				
	Lunch				
	Dinner				
	Night				

Sunday		Before	After	Dose	Notes
	Breakfast				
	Lunch				
	Dinner				
	Night				

Notes _____
_____
_____
_____
_____
_____
_____
_____
_____
_____
_____

Start of week date _____

Monday		Before	After	Dose	Notes
	Breakfast				
	Lunch				
	Dinner				
	Night				

Tuesday		Before	After	Dose	Notes
	Breakfast				
	Lunch				
	Dinner				
	Night				

Wednesday		Before	After	Dose	Notes
	Breakfast				
	Lunch				
	Dinner				
	Night				

Thursday		Before	After	Dose	Notes
	Breakfast				
	Lunch				
	Dinner				
	Night				

Notes _____

_____

_____

_____

Friday		Before	After	Dose	Notes
	Breakfast				
	Lunch				
	Dinner				
	Night				

Saturday		Before	After	Dose	Notes
	Breakfast				
	Lunch				
	Dinner				
	Night				

Sunday		Before	After	Dose	Notes
	Breakfast				
	Lunch				
	Dinner				
	Night				

Notes _____

_____

_____

_____

_____

_____

_____

_____

_____

_____

_____

Start of week date _____

Monday		Before	After	Dose	Notes
	Breakfast				
	Lunch				
	Dinner				
	Night				

Tuesday		Before	After	Dose	Notes
	Breakfast				
	Lunch				
	Dinner				
	Night				

Wednesday		Before	After	Dose	Notes
	Breakfast				
	Lunch				
	Dinner				
	Night				

Thursday		Before	After	Dose	Notes
	Breakfast				
	Lunch				
	Dinner				
	Night				

Notes _____
_____
_____
_____

Friday		Before	After	Dose	Notes
	Breakfast				
	Lunch				
	Dinner				
	Night				

Saturday		Before	After	Dose	Notes
	Breakfast				
	Lunch				
	Dinner				
	Night				

Sunday		Before	After	Dose	Notes
	Breakfast				
	Lunch				
	Dinner				
	Night				

Notes _____
_____
_____
_____
_____
_____
_____
_____
_____
_____
_____
_____

Start of week date _____

Monday		Before	After	Dose	Notes
	Breakfast				
	Lunch				
	Dinner				
	Night				

Tuesday		Before	After	Dose	Notes
	Breakfast				
	Lunch				
	Dinner				
	Night				

Wednesday		Before	After	Dose	Notes
	Breakfast				
	Lunch				
	Dinner				
	Night				

Thursday		Before	After	Dose	Notes
	Breakfast				
	Lunch				
	Dinner				
	Night				

Notes _____

_____

_____

_____

Friday		Before	After	Dose	Notes
	Breakfast				
	Lunch				
	Dinner				
	Night				

Saturday		Before	After	Dose	Notes
	Breakfast				
	Lunch				
	Dinner				
	Night				

Sunday		Before	After	Dose	Notes
	Breakfast				
	Lunch				
	Dinner				
	Night				

Notes _____

_____

_____

_____

_____

_____

_____

_____

_____

_____

_____

Start of week date _____

Monday		Before	After	Dose	Notes
	Breakfast				
	Lunch				
	Dinner				
	Night				

Tuesday		Before	After	Dose	Notes
	Breakfast				
	Lunch				
	Dinner				
	Night				

Wednesday		Before	After	Dose	Notes
	Breakfast				
	Lunch				
	Dinner				
	Night				

Thursday		Before	After	Dose	Notes
	Breakfast				
	Lunch				
	Dinner				
	Night				

Notes _____

_____

_____

_____

Friday		Before	After	Dose	Notes
	Breakfast				
	Lunch				
	Dinner				
	Night				

Saturday		Before	After	Dose	Notes
	Breakfast				
	Lunch				
	Dinner				
	Night				

Sunday		Before	After	Dose	Notes
	Breakfast				
	Lunch				
	Dinner				
	Night				

Notes _____

_____
_____
_____
_____
_____
_____
_____
_____
_____
_____

Start of week date _____

Monday		Before	After	Dose	Notes
	Breakfast				
	Lunch				
	Dinner				
	Night				

Tuesday		Before	After	Dose	Notes
	Breakfast				
	Lunch				
	Dinner				
	Night				

Wednesday		Before	After	Dose	Notes
	Breakfast				
	Lunch				
	Dinner				
	Night				

Thursday		Before	After	Dose	Notes
	Breakfast				
	Lunch				
	Dinner				
	Night				

Notes _____

_____

_____

_____

Friday		Before	After	Dose	Notes
	Breakfast				
	Lunch				
	Dinner				
	Night				

Saturday		Before	After	Dose	Notes
	Breakfast				
	Lunch				
	Dinner				
	Night				

Sunday		Before	After	Dose	Notes
	Breakfast				
	Lunch				
	Dinner				
	Night				

Notes _____

_____
_____
_____
_____
_____
_____
_____
_____
_____
_____
_____

Start of week date _____

Monday		Before	After	Dose	Notes
	Breakfast				
	Lunch				
	Dinner				
	Night				

Tuesday		Before	After	Dose	Notes
	Breakfast				
	Lunch				
	Dinner				
	Night				

Wednesday		Before	After	Dose	Notes
	Breakfast				
	Lunch				
	Dinner				
	Night				

Thursday		Before	After	Dose	Notes
	Breakfast				
	Lunch				
	Dinner				
	Night				

Notes _____

_____

_____

_____

Friday		Before	After	Dose	Notes
	Breakfast				
	Lunch				
	Dinner				
	Night				

Saturday		Before	After	Dose	Notes
	Breakfast				
	Lunch				
	Dinner				
	Night				

Sunday		Before	After	Dose	Notes
	Breakfast				
	Lunch				
	Dinner				
	Night				

Notes _____

_____

_____

_____

_____

_____

_____

_____

_____

_____

_____

_____

Start of week date _____

Monday		Before	After	Dose	Notes
	Breakfast				
	Lunch				
	Dinner				
	Night				

Tuesday		Before	After	Dose	Notes
	Breakfast				
	Lunch				
	Dinner				
	Night				

Wednesday		Before	After	Dose	Notes
	Breakfast				
	Lunch				
	Dinner				
	Night				

Thursday		Before	After	Dose	Notes
	Breakfast				
	Lunch				
	Dinner				
	Night				

Notes _____

_____

_____

_____

Friday		Before	After	Dose	Notes
	Breakfast				
	Lunch				
	Dinner				
	Night				

Saturday		Before	After	Dose	Notes
	Breakfast				
	Lunch				
	Dinner				
	Night				

Sunday		Before	After	Dose	Notes
	Breakfast				
	Lunch				
	Dinner				
	Night				

Notes _____

_____

_____

_____

_____

_____

_____

_____

_____

_____

_____

Start of week date _____

Monday		Before	After	Dose	Notes
	Breakfast				
	Lunch				
	Dinner				
	Night				

Tuesday		Before	After	Dose	Notes
	Breakfast				
	Lunch				
	Dinner				
	Night				

Wednesday		Before	After	Dose	Notes
	Breakfast				
	Lunch				
	Dinner				
	Night				

Thursday		Before	After	Dose	Notes
	Breakfast				
	Lunch				
	Dinner				
	Night				

Notes _____

_____

_____

_____

Friday		Before	After	Dose	Notes
	Breakfast				
	Lunch				
	Dinner				
	Night				

Saturday		Before	After	Dose	Notes
	Breakfast				
	Lunch				
	Dinner				
	Night				

Sunday		Before	After	Dose	Notes
	Breakfast				
	Lunch				
	Dinner				
	Night				

Notes _____

_____

_____

_____

_____

_____

_____

_____

_____

_____

_____

Start of week date _____

Monday		Before	After	Dose	Notes
	Breakfast				
	Lunch				
	Dinner				
	Night				

Tuesday		Before	After	Dose	Notes
	Breakfast				
	Lunch				
	Dinner				
	Night				

Wednesday		Before	After	Dose	Notes
	Breakfast				
	Lunch				
	Dinner				
	Night				

Thursday		Before	After	Dose	Notes
	Breakfast				
	Lunch				
	Dinner				
	Night				

Notes _____

Friday		Before	After	Dose	Notes
	Breakfast				
	Lunch				
	Dinner				
	Night				

Saturday		Before	After	Dose	Notes
	Breakfast				
	Lunch				
	Dinner				
	Night				

Sunday		Before	After	Dose	Notes
	Breakfast				
	Lunch				
	Dinner				
	Night				

Notes _____
_____
_____
_____
_____
_____
_____
_____
_____
_____
_____
_____

Start of week date _____

Monday		Before	After	Dose	Notes
	Breakfast				
	Lunch				
	Dinner				
	Night				

Tuesday		Before	After	Dose	Notes
	Breakfast				
	Lunch				
	Dinner				
	Night				

Wednesday		Before	After	Dose	Notes
	Breakfast				
	Lunch				
	Dinner				
	Night				

Thursday		Before	After	Dose	Notes
	Breakfast				
	Lunch				
	Dinner				
	Night				

Notes _____
_____
_____
_____

Friday		Before	After	Dose	Notes
	Breakfast				
	Lunch				
	Dinner				
	Night				

Saturday		Before	After	Dose	Notes
	Breakfast				
	Lunch				
	Dinner				
	Night				

Sunday		Before	After	Dose	Notes
	Breakfast				
	Lunch				
	Dinner				
	Night				

Notes _____
_____
_____
_____
_____
_____
_____
_____
_____
_____
_____

Start of week date _____

Monday		Before	After	Dose	Notes
	Breakfast				
	Lunch				
	Dinner				
	Night				

Tuesday		Before	After	Dose	Notes
	Breakfast				
	Lunch				
	Dinner				
	Night				

Wednesday		Before	After	Dose	Notes
	Breakfast				
	Lunch				
	Dinner				
	Night				

Thursday		Before	After	Dose	Notes
	Breakfast				
	Lunch				
	Dinner				
	Night				

Notes _____

_____

_____

_____

Friday		Before	After	Dose	Notes
	Breakfast				
	Lunch				
	Dinner				
	Night				

Saturday		Before	After	Dose	Notes
	Breakfast				
	Lunch				
	Dinner				
	Night				

Sunday		Before	After	Dose	Notes
	Breakfast				
	Lunch				
	Dinner				
	Night				

Notes _____
_____
_____
_____
_____
_____
_____
_____
_____
_____
_____
_____

Start of week date _____

Monday		Before	After	Dose	Notes
	Breakfast				
	Lunch				
	Dinner				
	Night				

Tuesday		Before	After	Dose	Notes
	Breakfast				
	Lunch				
	Dinner				
	Night				

Wednesday		Before	After	Dose	Notes
	Breakfast				
	Lunch				
	Dinner				
	Night				

Thursday		Before	After	Dose	Notes
	Breakfast				
	Lunch				
	Dinner				
	Night				

Notes _____

_____

_____

Friday		Before	After	Dose	Notes
	Breakfast				
	Lunch				
	Dinner				
	Night				

Saturday		Before	After	Dose	Notes
	Breakfast				
	Lunch				
	Dinner				
	Night				

Sunday		Before	After	Dose	Notes
	Breakfast				
	Lunch				
	Dinner				
	Night				

Notes _____
_____
_____
_____
_____
_____
_____
_____
_____
_____
_____

Start of week date _____

Monday		Before	After	Dose	Notes
	Breakfast				
	Lunch				
	Dinner				
	Night				

Tuesday		Before	After	Dose	Notes
	Breakfast				
	Lunch				
	Dinner				
	Night				

Wednesday		Before	After	Dose	Notes
	Breakfast				
	Lunch				
	Dinner				
	Night				

Thursday		Before	After	Dose	Notes
	Breakfast				
	Lunch				
	Dinner				
	Night				

Notes _____

_____

_____

Friday		Before	After	Dose	Notes
	Breakfast				
	Lunch				
	Dinner				
	Night				

Saturday		Before	After	Dose	Notes
	Breakfast				
	Lunch				
	Dinner				
	Night				

Sunday		Before	After	Dose	Notes
	Breakfast				
	Lunch				
	Dinner				
	Night				

Notes _____

_____

_____

_____

_____

_____

_____

_____

_____

_____

_____

Start of week date _____

Monday		Before	After	Dose	Notes
	Breakfast				
	Lunch				
	Dinner				
	Night				

Tuesday		Before	After	Dose	Notes
	Breakfast				
	Lunch				
	Dinner				
	Night				

Wednesday		Before	After	Dose	Notes
	Breakfast				
	Lunch				
	Dinner				
	Night				

Thursday		Before	After	Dose	Notes
	Breakfast				
	Lunch				
	Dinner				
	Night				

Notes _____

_____

_____

_____

Friday		Before	After	Dose	Notes
	Breakfast				
	Lunch				
	Dinner				
	Night				

Saturday		Before	After	Dose	Notes
	Breakfast				
	Lunch				
	Dinner				
	Night				

Sunday		Before	After	Dose	Notes
	Breakfast				
	Lunch				
	Dinner				
	Night				

Notes _____

_____
_____
_____
_____
_____
_____
_____
_____
_____
_____

Start of week date _____

Monday		Before	After	Dose	Notes
	Breakfast				
	Lunch				
	Dinner				
	Night				

Tuesday		Before	After	Dose	Notes
	Breakfast				
	Lunch				
	Dinner				
	Night				

Wednesday		Before	After	Dose	Notes
	Breakfast				
	Lunch				
	Dinner				
	Night				

Thursday		Before	After	Dose	Notes
	Breakfast				
	Lunch				
	Dinner				
	Night				

Notes _____

_____

_____

_____

Friday		Before	After	Dose	Notes
	Breakfast				
	Lunch				
	Dinner				
	Night				

Saturday		Before	After	Dose	Notes
	Breakfast				
	Lunch				
	Dinner				
	Night				

Sunday		Before	After	Dose	Notes
	Breakfast				
	Lunch				
	Dinner				
	Night				

Notes _____
_____
_____
_____
_____
_____
_____
_____
_____
_____
_____

Start of week date _____

Monday		Before	After	Dose	Notes
	Breakfast				
	Lunch				
	Dinner				
	Night				

Tuesday		Before	After	Dose	Notes
	Breakfast				
	Lunch				
	Dinner				
	Night				

Wednesday		Before	After	Dose	Notes
	Breakfast				
	Lunch				
	Dinner				
	Night				

Thursday		Before	After	Dose	Notes
	Breakfast				
	Lunch				
	Dinner				
	Night				

Notes _____

_____

_____

_____

Friday		Before	After	Dose	Notes
	Breakfast				
	Lunch				
	Dinner				
	Night				

Saturday		Before	After	Dose	Notes
	Breakfast				
	Lunch				
	Dinner				
	Night				

Sunday		Before	After	Dose	Notes
	Breakfast				
	Lunch				
	Dinner				
	Night				

Notes _____

_____

_____

_____

_____

_____

_____

_____

_____

_____

_____

Start of week date _____

Monday		Before	After	Dose	Notes
	Breakfast				
	Lunch				
	Dinner				
	Night				

Tuesday		Before	After	Dose	Notes
	Breakfast				
	Lunch				
	Dinner				
	Night				

Wednesday		Before	After	Dose	Notes
	Breakfast				
	Lunch				
	Dinner				
	Night				

Thursday		Before	After	Dose	Notes
	Breakfast				
	Lunch				
	Dinner				
	Night				

Notes _____

_____

_____

_____

Friday		Before	After	Dose	Notes
	Breakfast				
	Lunch				
	Dinner				
	Night				

Saturday		Before	After	Dose	Notes
	Breakfast				
	Lunch				
	Dinner				
	Night				

Sunday		Before	After	Dose	Notes
	Breakfast				
	Lunch				
	Dinner				
	Night				

Notes _____

_____

_____

_____

_____

_____

_____

_____

_____

_____

_____

_____

Start of week date _____

Monday		Before	After	Dose	Notes
	Breakfast				
	Lunch				
	Dinner				
	Night				

Tuesday		Before	After	Dose	Notes
	Breakfast				
	Lunch				
	Dinner				
	Night				

Wednesday		Before	After	Dose	Notes
	Breakfast				
	Lunch				
	Dinner				
	Night				

Thursday		Before	After	Dose	Notes
	Breakfast				
	Lunch				
	Dinner				
	Night				

Notes _____
_____
_____
_____

Friday		Before	After	Dose	Notes
	Breakfast				
	Lunch				
	Dinner				
	Night				

Saturday		Before	After	Dose	Notes
	Breakfast				
	Lunch				
	Dinner				
	Night				

Sunday		Before	After	Dose	Notes
	Breakfast				
	Lunch				
	Dinner				
	Night				

Notes _____
_____
_____
_____
_____
_____
_____
_____
_____
_____
_____
_____

Start of week date _____

Monday		Before	After	Dose	Notes
	Breakfast				
	Lunch				
	Dinner				
	Night				

Tuesday		Before	After	Dose	Notes
	Breakfast				
	Lunch				
	Dinner				
	Night				

Wednesday		Before	After	Dose	Notes
	Breakfast				
	Lunch				
	Dinner				
	Night				

Thursday		Before	After	Dose	Notes
	Breakfast				
	Lunch				
	Dinner				
	Night				

Notes _____

_____

_____

Friday		Before	After	Dose	Notes
	Breakfast				
	Lunch				
	Dinner				
	Night				

Saturday		Before	After	Dose	Notes
	Breakfast				
	Lunch				
	Dinner				
	Night				

Sunday		Before	After	Dose	Notes
	Breakfast				
	Lunch				
	Dinner				
	Night				

Notes _____
_____
_____
_____
_____
_____
_____
_____
_____
_____
_____
_____

Start of week date _____

Monday		Before	After	Dose	Notes
	Breakfast				
	Lunch				
	Dinner				
	Night				

Tuesday		Before	After	Dose	Notes
	Breakfast				
	Lunch				
	Dinner				
	Night				

Wednesday		Before	After	Dose	Notes
	Breakfast				
	Lunch				
	Dinner				
	Night				

Thursday		Before	After	Dose	Notes
	Breakfast				
	Lunch				
	Dinner				
	Night				

Notes _____

_____

_____

_____

Friday		Before	After	Dose	Notes
	Breakfast				
	Lunch				
	Dinner				
	Night				

Saturday		Before	After	Dose	Notes
	Breakfast				
	Lunch				
	Dinner				
	Night				

Sunday		Before	After	Dose	Notes
	Breakfast				
	Lunch				
	Dinner				
	Night				

Notes _____

_____

_____

_____

_____

_____

_____

_____

_____

_____

_____

Start of week date _____

Monday		Before	After	Dose	Notes
	Breakfast				
	Lunch				
	Dinner				
	Night				

Tuesday		Before	After	Dose	Notes
	Breakfast				
	Lunch				
	Dinner				
	Night				

Wednesday		Before	After	Dose	Notes
	Breakfast				
	Lunch				
	Dinner				
	Night				

Thursday		Before	After	Dose	Notes
	Breakfast				
	Lunch				
	Dinner				
	Night				

Notes _____
_____
_____
_____

Friday		Before	After	Dose	Notes
	Breakfast				
	Lunch				
	Dinner				
	Night				

Saturday		Before	After	Dose	Notes
	Breakfast				
	Lunch				
	Dinner				
	Night				

Sunday		Before	After	Dose	Notes
	Breakfast				
	Lunch				
	Dinner				
	Night				

Notes _____
_____
_____
_____
_____
_____
_____
_____
_____
_____
_____

Start of week date _____

Monday		Before	After	Dose	Notes
	Breakfast				
	Lunch				
	Dinner				
	Night				

Tuesday		Before	After	Dose	Notes
	Breakfast				
	Lunch				
	Dinner				
	Night				

Wednesday		Before	After	Dose	Notes
	Breakfast				
	Lunch				
	Dinner				
	Night				

Thursday		Before	After	Dose	Notes
	Breakfast				
	Lunch				
	Dinner				
	Night				

Notes _____

_____

_____

_____

Friday		Before	After	Dose	Notes
	Breakfast				
	Lunch				
	Dinner				
	Night				

Saturday		Before	After	Dose	Notes
	Breakfast				
	Lunch				
	Dinner				
	Night				

Sunday		Before	After	Dose	Notes
	Breakfast				
	Lunch				
	Dinner				
	Night				

Notes _____

_____

_____

_____

_____

_____

_____

_____

_____

_____

_____

_____

Start of week date _____

Monday		Before	After	Dose	Notes
	Breakfast				
	Lunch				
	Dinner				
	Night				

Tuesday		Before	After	Dose	Notes
	Breakfast				
	Lunch				
	Dinner				
	Night				

Wednesday		Before	After	Dose	Notes
	Breakfast				
	Lunch				
	Dinner				
	Night				

Thursday		Before	After	Dose	Notes
	Breakfast				
	Lunch				
	Dinner				
	Night				

Notes _____

_____

_____

_____

Friday		Before	After	Dose	Notes
	Breakfast				
	Lunch				
	Dinner				
	Night				

Saturday		Before	After	Dose	Notes
	Breakfast				
	Lunch				
	Dinner				
	Night				

Sunday		Before	After	Dose	Notes
	Breakfast				
	Lunch				
	Dinner				
	Night				

Notes _____

_____
_____
_____
_____
_____
_____
_____
_____
_____
_____
_____

Start of week date _____

		Before	After	Dose	Notes
Monday	Breakfast				
	Lunch				
	Dinner				
	Night				

		Before	After	Dose	Notes
Tuesday	Breakfast				
	Lunch				
	Dinner				
	Night				

		Before	After	Dose	Notes
Wednesday	Breakfast				
	Lunch				
	Dinner				
	Night				

		Before	After	Dose	Notes
Thursday	Breakfast				
	Lunch				
	Dinner				
	Night				

Notes _____

_____

_____

_____

Friday		Before	After	Dose	Notes
	Breakfast				
	Lunch				
	Dinner				
	Night				

Saturday		Before	After	Dose	Notes
	Breakfast				
	Lunch				
	Dinner				
	Night				

Sunday		Before	After	Dose	Notes
	Breakfast				
	Lunch				
	Dinner				
	Night				

Notes _____
_____
_____
_____
_____
_____
_____
_____
_____
_____
_____

Start of week date _____

Monday		Before	After	Dose	Notes
	Breakfast				
	Lunch				
	Dinner				
	Night				

Tuesday		Before	After	Dose	Notes
	Breakfast				
	Lunch				
	Dinner				
	Night				

Wednesday		Before	After	Dose	Notes
	Breakfast				
	Lunch				
	Dinner				
	Night				

Thursday		Before	After	Dose	Notes
	Breakfast				
	Lunch				
	Dinner				
	Night				

Notes _____
_____
_____
_____

Friday		Before	After	Dose	Notes
	Breakfast				
	Lunch				
	Dinner				
	Night				

Saturday		Before	After	Dose	Notes
	Breakfast				
	Lunch				
	Dinner				
	Night				

Sunday		Before	After	Dose	Notes
	Breakfast				
	Lunch				
	Dinner				
	Night				

Notes _____

_____

_____

_____

_____

_____

_____

_____

_____

_____

_____

Start of week date _____

Monday		Before	After	Dose	Notes
	Breakfast				
	Lunch				
	Dinner				
	Night				

Tuesday		Before	After	Dose	Notes
	Breakfast				
	Lunch				
	Dinner				
	Night				

Wednesday		Before	After	Dose	Notes
	Breakfast				
	Lunch				
	Dinner				
	Night				

Thursday		Before	After	Dose	Notes
	Breakfast				
	Lunch				
	Dinner				
	Night				

Notes _____

_____

_____

_____

Friday		Before	After	Dose	Notes
	Breakfast				
	Lunch				
	Dinner				
	Night				

Saturday		Before	After	Dose	Notes
	Breakfast				
	Lunch				
	Dinner				
	Night				

Sunday		Before	After	Dose	Notes
	Breakfast				
	Lunch				
	Dinner				
	Night				

Notes _____
_____
_____
_____
_____
_____
_____
_____
_____
_____
_____
_____

Start of week date _____

Monday		Before	After	Dose	Notes
	Breakfast				
	Lunch				
	Dinner				
	Night				

Tuesday		Before	After	Dose	Notes
	Breakfast				
	Lunch				
	Dinner				
	Night				

Wednesday		Before	After	Dose	Notes
	Breakfast				
	Lunch				
	Dinner				
	Night				

Thursday		Before	After	Dose	Notes
	Breakfast				
	Lunch				
	Dinner				
	Night				

Notes _____
_____
_____
_____

Friday		Before	After	Dose	Notes
	Breakfast				
	Lunch				
	Dinner				
	Night				

Saturday		Before	After	Dose	Notes
	Breakfast				
	Lunch				
	Dinner				
	Night				

Sunday		Before	After	Dose	Notes
	Breakfast				
	Lunch				
	Dinner				
	Night				

Notes _____
_____
_____
_____
_____
_____
_____
_____
_____
_____
_____

Start of week date _____

Monday		Before	After	Dose	Notes
	Breakfast				
	Lunch				
	Dinner				
	Night				

Tuesday		Before	After	Dose	Notes
	Breakfast				
	Lunch				
	Dinner				
	Night				

Wednesday		Before	After	Dose	Notes
	Breakfast				
	Lunch				
	Dinner				
	Night				

Thursday		Before	After	Dose	Notes
	Breakfast				
	Lunch				
	Dinner				
	Night				

Notes _____
_____
_____
_____

Friday		Before	After	Dose	Notes
	Breakfast				
	Lunch				
	Dinner				
	Night				

Saturday		Before	After	Dose	Notes
	Breakfast				
	Lunch				
	Dinner				
	Night				

Sunday		Before	After	Dose	Notes
	Breakfast				
	Lunch				
	Dinner				
	Night				

Notes _____

_____

_____

_____

_____

_____

_____

_____

_____

_____

_____

Start of week date _____

Monday		Before	After	Dose	Notes
	Breakfast				
	Lunch				
	Dinner				
	Night				

Tuesday		Before	After	Dose	Notes
	Breakfast				
	Lunch				
	Dinner				
	Night				

Wednesday		Before	After	Dose	Notes
	Breakfast				
	Lunch				
	Dinner				
	Night				

Thursday		Before	After	Dose	Notes
	Breakfast				
	Lunch				
	Dinner				
	Night				

Notes _____

_____

_____

_____

Friday		Before	After	Dose	Notes
	Breakfast				
	Lunch				
	Dinner				
	Night				

Saturday		Before	After	Dose	Notes
	Breakfast				
	Lunch				
	Dinner				
	Night				

Sunday		Before	After	Dose	Notes
	Breakfast				
	Lunch				
	Dinner				
	Night				

Notes _____
_____
_____
_____
_____
_____
_____
_____
_____
_____
_____
_____

Start of week date _____

Monday		Before	After	Dose	Notes
	Breakfast				
	Lunch				
	Dinner				
	Night				

Tuesday		Before	After	Dose	Notes
	Breakfast				
	Lunch				
	Dinner				
	Night				

Wednesday		Before	After	Dose	Notes
	Breakfast				
	Lunch				
	Dinner				
	Night				

Thursday		Before	After	Dose	Notes
	Breakfast				
	Lunch				
	Dinner				
	Night				

Notes _____

_____

_____

_____

Friday		Before	After	Dose	Notes
	Breakfast				
	Lunch				
	Dinner				
	Night				

Saturday		Before	After	Dose	Notes
	Breakfast				
	Lunch				
	Dinner				
	Night				

Sunday		Before	After	Dose	Notes
	Breakfast				
	Lunch				
	Dinner				
	Night				

Notes _____

_____
_____
_____
_____
_____
_____
_____
_____
_____
_____

Start of week date _____

Monday		Before	After	Dose	Notes
	Breakfast				
	Lunch				
	Dinner				
	Night				

Tuesday		Before	After	Dose	Notes
	Breakfast				
	Lunch				
	Dinner				
	Night				

Wednesday		Before	After	Dose	Notes
	Breakfast				
	Lunch				
	Dinner				
	Night				

Thursday		Before	After	Dose	Notes
	Breakfast				
	Lunch				
	Dinner				
	Night				

Notes _____
_____
_____
_____

Friday		Before	After	Dose	Notes
	Breakfast				
	Lunch				
	Dinner				
	Night				

Saturday		Before	After	Dose	Notes
	Breakfast				
	Lunch				
	Dinner				
	Night				

Sunday		Before	After	Dose	Notes
	Breakfast				
	Lunch				
	Dinner				
	Night				

Notes _____

_____

_____

_____

_____

_____

_____

_____

_____

_____

_____

_____

Start of week date _____

Monday		Before	After	Dose	Notes
	Breakfast				
	Lunch				
	Dinner				
	Night				

Tuesday		Before	After	Dose	Notes
	Breakfast				
	Lunch				
	Dinner				
	Night				

Wednesday		Before	After	Dose	Notes
	Breakfast				
	Lunch				
	Dinner				
	Night				

Thursday		Before	After	Dose	Notes
	Breakfast				
	Lunch				
	Dinner				
	Night				

Notes _____

_____

_____

_____

Friday		Before	After	Dose	Notes
	Breakfast				
	Lunch				
	Dinner				
	Night				

Saturday		Before	After	Dose	Notes
	Breakfast				
	Lunch				
	Dinner				
	Night				

Sunday		Before	After	Dose	Notes
	Breakfast				
	Lunch				
	Dinner				
	Night				

Notes _____

_____

_____

_____

_____

_____

_____

_____

_____

_____

_____

Start of week date _____

Monday		Before	After	Dose	Notes
	Breakfast				
	Lunch				
	Dinner				
	Night				

Tuesday		Before	After	Dose	Notes
	Breakfast				
	Lunch				
	Dinner				
	Night				

Wednesday		Before	After	Dose	Notes
	Breakfast				
	Lunch				
	Dinner				
	Night				

Thursday		Before	After	Dose	Notes
	Breakfast				
	Lunch				
	Dinner				
	Night				

Notes _____

_____

_____

_____

Friday		Before	After	Dose	Notes
	Breakfast				
	Lunch				
	Dinner				
	Night				

Saturday		Before	After	Dose	Notes
	Breakfast				
	Lunch				
	Dinner				
	Night				

Sunday		Before	After	Dose	Notes
	Breakfast				
	Lunch				
	Dinner				
	Night				

Notes _____

_____

_____

_____

_____

_____

_____

_____

_____

_____

_____

Start of week date _____

Monday		Before	After	Dose	Notes
	Breakfast				
	Lunch				
	Dinner				
	Night				

Tuesday		Before	After	Dose	Notes
	Breakfast				
	Lunch				
	Dinner				
	Night				

Wednesday		Before	After	Dose	Notes
	Breakfast				
	Lunch				
	Dinner				
	Night				

Thursday		Before	After	Dose	Notes
	Breakfast				
	Lunch				
	Dinner				
	Night				

Notes _____

_____

_____

_____

Friday		Before	After	Dose	Notes
	Breakfast				
	Lunch				
	Dinner				
	Night				

Saturday		Before	After	Dose	Notes
	Breakfast				
	Lunch				
	Dinner				
	Night				

Sunday		Before	After	Dose	Notes
	Breakfast				
	Lunch				
	Dinner				
	Night				

Notes _____
_____
_____
_____
_____
_____
_____
_____
_____
_____
_____

Start of week date _____

Monday		Before	After	Dose	Notes
	Breakfast				
	Lunch				
	Dinner				
	Night				

Tuesday		Before	After	Dose	Notes
	Breakfast				
	Lunch				
	Dinner				
	Night				

Wednesday		Before	After	Dose	Notes
	Breakfast				
	Lunch				
	Dinner				
	Night				

Thursday		Before	After	Dose	Notes
	Breakfast				
	Lunch				
	Dinner				
	Night				

Notes _____

_____

_____

_____

Friday		Before	After	Dose	Notes
	Breakfast				
	Lunch				
	Dinner				
	Night				

Saturday		Before	After	Dose	Notes
	Breakfast				
	Lunch				
	Dinner				
	Night				

Sunday		Before	After	Dose	Notes
	Breakfast				
	Lunch				
	Dinner				
	Night				

Notes _____
_____
_____
_____
_____
_____
_____
_____
_____
_____
_____
_____

Start of week date _____

Monday		Before	After	Dose	Notes
	Breakfast				
	Lunch				
	Dinner				
	Night				

Tuesday		Before	After	Dose	Notes
	Breakfast				
	Lunch				
	Dinner				
	Night				

Wednesday		Before	After	Dose	Notes
	Breakfast				
	Lunch				
	Dinner				
	Night				

Thursday		Before	After	Dose	Notes
	Breakfast				
	Lunch				
	Dinner				
	Night				

Notes _____

_____
_____
_____

Friday		Before	After	Dose	Notes
	Breakfast				
	Lunch				
	Dinner				
	Night				

Saturday		Before	After	Dose	Notes
	Breakfast				
	Lunch				
	Dinner				
	Night				

Sunday		Before	After	Dose	Notes
	Breakfast				
	Lunch				
	Dinner				
	Night				

Notes _____

_____

_____

_____

_____

_____

_____

_____

_____

_____

_____

_____

Start of week date _____

Monday		Before	After	Dose	Notes
	Breakfast				
	Lunch				
	Dinner				
	Night				

Tuesday		Before	After	Dose	Notes
	Breakfast				
	Lunch				
	Dinner				
	Night				

Wednesday		Before	After	Dose	Notes
	Breakfast				
	Lunch				
	Dinner				
	Night				

Thursday		Before	After	Dose	Notes
	Breakfast				
	Lunch				
	Dinner				
	Night				

Notes _____

_____

_____

_____

Friday		Before	After	Dose	Notes
	Breakfast				
	Lunch				
	Dinner				
	Night				

Saturday		Before	After	Dose	Notes
	Breakfast				
	Lunch				
	Dinner				
	Night				

Sunday		Before	After	Dose	Notes
	Breakfast				
	Lunch				
	Dinner				
	Night				

Notes _____
_____
_____
_____
_____
_____
_____
_____
_____
_____
_____
_____

Start of week date _____

Monday		Before	After	Dose	Notes
	Breakfast				
	Lunch				
	Dinner				
	Night				

Tuesday		Before	After	Dose	Notes
	Breakfast				
	Lunch				
	Dinner				
	Night				

Wednesday		Before	After	Dose	Notes
	Breakfast				
	Lunch				
	Dinner				
	Night				

Thursday		Before	After	Dose	Notes
	Breakfast				
	Lunch				
	Dinner				
	Night				

Notes _____

_____

_____

Friday		Before	After	Dose	Notes
	Breakfast				
	Lunch				
	Dinner				
	Night				

Saturday		Before	After	Dose	Notes
	Breakfast				
	Lunch				
	Dinner				
	Night				

Sunday		Before	After	Dose	Notes
	Breakfast				
	Lunch				
	Dinner				
	Night				

Notes _____
_____
_____
_____
_____
_____
_____
_____
_____
_____
_____

Start of week date _____

Monday		Before	After	Dose	Notes
	Breakfast				
	Lunch				
	Dinner				
	Night				

Tuesday		Before	After	Dose	Notes
	Breakfast				
	Lunch				
	Dinner				
	Night				

Wednesday		Before	After	Dose	Notes
	Breakfast				
	Lunch				
	Dinner				
	Night				

Thursday		Before	After	Dose	Notes
	Breakfast				
	Lunch				
	Dinner				
	Night				

Notes _____

_____

_____

_____

Friday		Before	After	Dose	Notes
	Breakfast				
	Lunch				
	Dinner				
	Night				

Saturday		Before	After	Dose	Notes
	Breakfast				
	Lunch				
	Dinner				
	Night				

Sunday		Before	After	Dose	Notes
	Breakfast				
	Lunch				
	Dinner				
	Night				

Notes _____

_____
_____
_____
_____
_____
_____
_____
_____
_____
_____

Start of week date _____

Monday		Before	After	Dose	Notes
	Breakfast				
	Lunch				
	Dinner				
	Night				

Tuesday		Before	After	Dose	Notes
	Breakfast				
	Lunch				
	Dinner				
	Night				

Wednesday		Before	After	Dose	Notes
	Breakfast				
	Lunch				
	Dinner				
	Night				

Thursday		Before	After	Dose	Notes
	Breakfast				
	Lunch				
	Dinner				
	Night				

Notes _____
_____
_____
_____

Friday		Before	After	Dose	Notes
	Breakfast				
	Lunch				
	Dinner				
	Night				

Saturday		Before	After	Dose	Notes
	Breakfast				
	Lunch				
	Dinner				
	Night				

Sunday		Before	After	Dose	Notes
	Breakfast				
	Lunch				
	Dinner				
	Night				

Notes _____

_____

_____

_____

_____

_____

_____

_____

_____

_____

_____

_____

Thank you!

We hope you enjoyed our book.

As a small publishing company, your feedback is very important to us.

Please let us know how you liked our book at:

whiteorangepublishing@gmail.com

Made in the USA
Las Vegas, NV
09 July 2024

92032412R00066